Distribution, publication, and copying in any form are prohibited and subject to damages.

TEN HYPNOSES

Copying, publishing, and sharing with third parties are only permitted with the written consent of the author. Please observe the notes on copyright and usage.

Distribution, publication, and copying in any form are prohibited and subject to damages.

Copying, publishing, and sharing with third parties are only permitted with the written consent of the author. Please observe the notes on copyright and usage.

Distribution, publication, and copying in any form are prohibited and subject to damages.

Ingo Michael Simon

TEN HYPNOSES

28

Tinnitus, Ear Noises

Copying, publishing, and sharing with third parties are only permitted with the written consent of the author. Please observe the notes on copyright and usage.

Distribution, publication, and copying in any form are prohibited and subject to damages.

© 2024 Ingo Michael Simon
All rights reserved.
Independently published
www.ingosimon.com

Important Notes for Urgent Attention:

The contents of this book are based on the practical experiences of the author with hypnosis applications and psychotherapy in a trance state. Although the author has strived for the utmost care, errors or misunderstandings in the presentation cannot be completely excluded. Therapeutic work with people and the application of hypnosis are solely the responsibility of the hypnotist. It cannot be ruled out that parts of this book may be misunderstood or that the application of a presented procedure may cause an undesirable reaction in the client. The author also assumes no co-responsibility if work with a client is carried out with reference to the statements in this book.

The Author:

Ingo Michael Simon studied psychology and education and is a hypnotherapist with practices in southwestern Germany and Switzerland. With the help of hypnosis-supported psychotherapy, he primarily treats people with persistent psychological conditions. His practice focuses on anxiety disorders, pathological compulsions, and psychosomatic illnesses. His therapeutic offerings mainly include classical and modern hypnosis applications and the dreamland therapy he developed himself.

Copying, publishing, and sharing with third parties are only permitted with the written consent of the author. Please observe the notes on copyright and usage.

Distribution, publication, and copying in any form are prohibited and subject to damages.

INTRODUCTION	6
COPYRIGHT AND USAGE	8
HYPNOSIS 1	10
HYPNOSIS 2	15
HYPNOSIS 3	19
HYPNOSIS 4	24
HYPNOSIS 5	29
HYPNOSIS 6	34
HYPNOSIS 7	39
HYPNOSIS 8	44
HYPNOSIS 9	50
HYPNOSIS 10	55
ALL TITLES IN THE SERIES	60

Copying, publishing, and sharing with third parties are only permitted with the written consent of the author. Please observe the notes on copyright and usage.

Distribution, publication, and copying in any form are prohibited and subject to damages.

Introduction

The series "Ten Hypnoses" is very well known in Germany, Austria, and Switzerland as a collection of texts for therapeutic work and is used by numerous psychotherapeutic practices, doctors, therapists, coaches, and other helping professionals. I am pleased to now be able to offer these texts in other countries as well.

Most therapists have their own methods for inducing and deepening trance as well as for exiting trance. Therefore, I have focused on the main part of the hypnosis. The texts in this book can be integrated as the main part into any hypnosis process. The texts in this collection use various hypnosis techniques. I will not explain these in detail, as I assume that users have the appropriate training. It is also not necessary to understand the exact structure or functioning of the different parts. The texts can simply be read aloud, and they will have their effect.

Decide for yourself which text best suits your client or patient at any given time. You can also combine passages from different texts. It is not about using all ten hypnoses in sequence. It is a selection of possibilities.

Copying, publishing, and sharing with third parties are only permitted with the written consent of the author. Please observe the notes on copyright and usage.

I want to emphasize that books cannot replace therapy. Psychotherapy or other therapeutic treatments involve much more. A careful diagnosis is the necessary basis for deciding on the use of methods, including whether hypnosis or one of my texts should be used. Even in this case, preparatory discussions, follow-up discussions during the session, and of course, a therapeutic concept for the sequence of sessions and the content approaches are essential parts of therapy. This cannot and should not be achieved with a collection of texts.

In any case, I wish you much success in your work and I am pleased if my text templates can contribute in a small way.

Ingo Michael Simon

Distribution, publication, and copying in any form are prohibited and subject to damages.

Copyright and Usage

Copying, publishing, and sharing with third parties is prohibited and only permitted with the written consent of the author. Please observe the following copyright and usage guidelines.

This work has been carefully crafted and created to the best of the author's knowledge and personal experience. It comprises text templates and application guidelines for professional hypnosis sessions. The author is a licensed psychotherapist with extensive experience in psychotherapy, coaching, and personal training using hypnotic techniques and methods. Nevertheless, the author and the publisher assume no liability for the accuracy of information, instructions, and advice, nor for any typographical errors. The author and publisher accept no responsibility or liability for the application of these texts and recommendations with clients or patients, nor for any potential consequences or unexpected reactions. It is expressly noted that the application of therapeutic and advisory techniques and formulations lies solely and entirely within the responsibility of the practitioner. This also applies to adherence to the

Copying, publishing, and sharing with third parties are only permitted with the written consent of the author. Please observe the notes on copyright and usage.

boundaries of legally regulated medical and therapeutic practices. The fact that a book containing action proposals is freely available for sale does not imply that its application with clients or patients is permitted for everyone.

Hypnosis 1

You have a clear goal... You want to eliminate the noises in your ear, to turn them off... You are determined to get rid of the noises in your ear, to reduce them as much as possible... This is possible, and there are two ways to achieve it... Either you manage to throw out the noises, to really end them... or you may not completely eliminate them, but instead, they become indifferent to you... Both options lead to the same outcome, however you approach it... whichever of these two paths succeeds, you will reach your goal... No more disturbing noises in the ear... never again disturbing noises in your ear... End the noises... Stop them... and this is indeed possible... You have made up your mind, and it actually works...

Now, it's time to make another important decision... so that it can succeed now... Simply decide on one of the two successful paths... either turning it off or neutralizing it... However you decide, you will achieve the same success... the end of disturbing noises in the ear... Isn't it amazing that today, you're already taking the first step towards initiating the end of these ear noises? ... And just as amazing and helpful is the fact that you have the power to do so, and you're using it today...

Your thoughts are focusing on new content and ignoring the noises in the ear... If it's not easy to get rid of the hissing and ringing, it is possible to neutralize these noises... You develop the thought that tells you... Noises in the ear are like wind and don't interest me at all... because it is precisely this thought that helps you... So, you focus entirely on this thought, because any thought that you think intensely changes your situation... becomes reality... So, you attune yourself to this special thought... and with that, you hear the noises in the ear less and less... You tell yourself... Noises in the ear are like wind and don't interest me at all... and then it's exactly like that, you overlook these noises...

Perhaps you know that your body follows all your thoughts and feelings... so your body also follows your new thought that tells it that noises in the ear don't matter to you at all... that they don't interest you at all... Noises in the ear are neutral... completely neutral... and when your body knows that these noises in the ear are unimportant, it relaxes and doesn't transmit them further... because without the body's reactions, we can't hear noises in the ear... Tinnitus needs the body's pathway... but your body knows that these noises are indifferent to you, so it never supports them again... and with that, they automatically become quieter and smaller...

Your feelings are also important... as soon as you feel strenuous emotions and tensions, the noises are louder, but when you come to rest inwardly and relax, they become quieter... but perhaps you've experienced that these ear noises are particularly disturbing in quiet moments... but that's not true, that's a misconception... because even in quietness, we are often more strained than we think because our very deep thoughts and feelings are still in motion... You change that now through true relaxation... through true relaxation deep inside you... When you are truly deeply relaxed and inwardly calm, the ear noises also become quieter, it can't be any other way... So, if you now hear less noise or they don't bother you as much, you feel that you are truly in inner peace... and if the noises still bother you a lot right now, you can relax even deeper... Relax and become calm, then the noises will also become quieter...

Now imagine how carefree your everyday life can be once the noises have become very quiet in everyday life... and imagine how easily you can shape your day once the noises have become quiet and don't bother you much anymore because you hardly notice them... Then you can imagine that you move through the day with ease and good humor... that you enjoy work just as much as breaks and even quiet and silence because then real silence occurs... Then your organism now adjusts to moving through the day just as easily and naturally... to already behaving as if the noises have completely passed... as if noises in the ear had never been... Everything goes smoothly and easily... You feel free, and you move freely, and everything inside you is calm... Everything inside you is calm and comfortable... and everything inside you remains calm and comfortable...

Today you have made an important decision... You have decided that the end of the ear noises has now come... and for that, you have integrated a special thought... Noises in the ear are like wind and don't interest me at all... and moreover, you have made this thought a truth... Noises in the ear are like wind and don't interest me at all... and that's why it always happens exactly as your thought says... Noises in the ear are like wind and don't interest me at all... and ear noises come to an end... Ear noises come to an end...

Hypnosis 2

You have understood that it is time to change your path, to stop the ear noises as quickly as possible... It is remarkable how well you manage to fully focus on this goal... the end of tinnitus...

That's why you have also decided to process everything that contributed to the occurrence of ear noises in the past... It is remarkable how well you manage to look deep inside and process the causes of the ear noises...

Yes, today you are already starting to deeply and honestly process all the connections of the ear noises, because this frees you already today... It is remarkable how well you succeed at this...

You have understood that your deep inner self can help you, and that's why you chose hypnosis to end the buzzing/ringing and be free... It is remarkable how well you manage to trust your deep inner self now...

So, you now allow your deep inner self to process and dissolve all conflicts and entanglements deep within, because by doing so, you will become calmer inside and out, and the buzzing/ringing will stop as if by itself... It is remarkable how well you manage to fully trust your deep inner self and feel that it actually resolves all conflicts and entanglements deep within for you... and the disturbing ear noises disappear as a result...

Yes, you allow your deep inner self right now to process all conflicts and entanglements deep within and thereby make the ear noises quieter and even stop them completely... It is remarkable how well you succeed at this...

You have understood that you will reach your goal more easily if you treat yourself respectfully and lovingly and direct your thoughts constructively... It is remarkable how well you manage to direct and steer your thoughts constructively, with respect and love...

So, you now decide to think and feel with respect and love... Yes, I trust my deep inner self because it can free me from tinnitus immediately... It is remarkable how well you manage to continue to trust your deep inner self and feel that it indeed helps you optimally in letting go of the disturbing noises...

Yes, you now direct your thoughts respectfully and lovingly to fully trust your deep inner self and fully support the internal processing... You now direct your thoughts respectfully and lovingly... It is remarkable how well you succeed at this...

Your deep inner self has understood that there is something deep within you that wants to be heard... Your deep inner self knows all the causes and connections, all unresolved and repressed conflicts that led to this inner signal of noises... It is remarkable how well your deep inner self manages to recognize and understand this...

Your deep inner self, therefore, immediately takes over the task of resolving and processing exactly these connections today for you and then letting them go... It is remarkable how quickly your deep inner self can complete this task... It is remarkable how well you and your deep inner self are working hand in hand...

Yes, your deep inner self is already processing all repressed conflicts in this minute, allowing them and accepting them, because that dissolves the tinnitus... thereby dissolving all disturbing impulses and you feel inner peace and healing silence... It is remarkable how well you can already feel inner silence...

You have understood that today is a day of real transformation, of liberation and constructive change... It is remarkable how well you manage to embrace this change...

Therefore, you continue to trust in the support of your deep inner self, which helps you today and in the future... It is remarkable how well you manage to trust your deep inner self even in your waking everyday life...

Yes, you trust your deep inner self completely... for the end of tinnitus and for true inner peace and silence... It is remarkable how quickly the end of ear noises is possible...

Hypnosis 3

Anchor Technique (Haptic Anchor, Post-Hypnotic)

An anchor (or trigger) is a stimulus that is meant to create a specific feeling or evoke a particular thought. It is essentially a signal that is perceived by the client and then triggers an internal process. The established anchor then replaces the suggestion. In everyday life, a client can use an anchor to trigger or establish a desired state, even without a trance state. Numerous stimuli can be used as anchors/triggers. I work with the following possibilities, which I also use in the series "Ten Hypnosis Sessions": physical anchors (clenching the hand, pressing the ball of the thumb...), visual anchors (symbols, word cards...), acoustic anchors (signal noises like phone ringing, melodies...), olfactory anchors (essential oils...), tactile anchors (comfort objects, talismans...). Additionally, I distinguish between perihypnotic and post-hypnotic anchors. Perihypnotic anchors are those primarily used during hypnosis, where the therapist establishes the anchor and then repeatedly triggers it as a supplement to suggestions and visualizations. Post-hypnotic anchors are mainly set up for the time after the session, so that the client can help themselves with it.

Today we want to train your body to make the ear noises quieter... quieter and quieter... until they eventually stop bothering you... until they have become so quiet that you no longer notice them... Your body can influence the noises... they are not always the same intensity... You know that... sometimes they are louder, sometimes quieter... When you are distracted, you hear them less, sometimes you don't hear them at all... but even when you focus on the noises in the ear, they fluctuate... There are always moments when the buzzing or hissing diminishes briefly or even stops... But it's enough if it just gets quieter for a short moment... Imagine you could tell your body to do this for you at the push of a button... You wonder how that works? ... Well, it's easier than you think, because we can work with an anchor... an anchor is like a button, like a trigger for something... and your anchor is supposed to make the ear noises quieter at the push of a button... a simple press that signals your body to make the noises quieter now... and once this button works, you can use it over and over again... press it again and again and experience that the noises in the ear really get quieter... because your body has learned this connection... For this, I will now give you a soft ball that you can squeeze well... It will be your anchor... it will be your button... and whenever you squeeze it, your body will make the ear noises quieter... However, it's important to press the ball at the right moment so that your body learns correctly to make the ear noises quieter... I will explain to you how to do it to make it succeed, and then you'll have time to practice it... here and today... in just a few minutes, everything will be learned, and your tinnitus-off switch will work...

Now the training can begin... Follow my words, focus entirely on them... and in the meantime, pay attention to the tinnitus... casually, you can hear it... and whenever it gets a bit quieter, just squeeze the ball briefly... You squeeze it whenever it gets quieter, and only then, so that your body really learns this connection and you can use your switch in everyday life...

... [Give the client a small soft ball that fits well in the hand. It's best to discuss the procedure before hypnosis so that the client knows what to do in trance. Demonstrate it once. Then it works easily in trance. Observe during hypnosis how often the client squeezes the ball. Just make a mark on a piece of paper each time. This way, after the session, you can show the client that there were some moments with quieter noises.] ...

... [Please briefly confirm each ball squeeze: ... Yes, you squeezed the ball, the tinnitus has become quieter ... or ... Well done, the tinnitus has become quieter...] ...

... Now pay attention to my words and the tinnitus in the background... and whenever you feel the noise gets quieter, just squeeze the ball briefly... just briefly, as a signal... your body learns this connection quickly, but today, only squeeze when you also notice that the noises have at least become a bit quieter... just a little quieter is enough... Let everything come to you and listen to my words, which cause your ear noises to become quieter from time to time and then squeeze the ball... but above all... Don't help me with it... Only squeeze the ball when the noises really become quieter... and they will get quieter over time... maybe just briefly... maybe multiple times and again and again... or they will become quieter gradually, that happens too... You feel it yourself... you can hear it... My words are very clear, but in the background is also the tinnitus... it remains there, behind my words... sometimes loud and sometimes really quieter... and when it's quieter, quieter than before, then just squeeze... Just squeeze the ball when it gets quieter... then and now the noise is at least a bit quieter, and then squeeze the ball...

So, your switch works... Your body has registered that you squeezed the ball every time the ear noises got quieter... and so a special connection has been established... pressing the ball and making the ear noises quieter... so you can also make the ear noises quieter in your waking everyday life... simply by pressing the ball because your body then remembers that this connection exists... press the ball... reduce the noises... press the ball... reduce the noises... it's that simple... really that simple... You can take the ball with you in everyday life and always have it handy... and when you need it... when you really need it because the ear noises are bothering you, then take the ball and squeeze it... and the noises will get quieter...

Hypnosis 4

Today is a special day because you want to end the annoying ear noises... You have tried many times, but so far, it hasn't worked... but today is different because today you are here to do it in trance... Many people believe that they are reprogrammed in trance... but that is not necessary at all because who should reprogram you... who should change something in you if not yourself... Perhaps there were some suggestions on what can be done to relieve ear noises, but today you are doing everything yourself... today you change your fundamental attitude, more precisely, the fundamental attitude of your subconscious mind towards the noises because you can influence your subconscious mind, your deep and unconscious attitudes... through very targeted thoughts... and that is what you do today... You send a targeted thought into your subconscious mind and thereby change the noises because they are only there on the surface... behind the noises, it is quiet...

In a few moments, it will begin... it is like a meditation where you come to rest to then find something new or to take a new path... in meditative rest, this is possible because our feeling can do more than our mind... and when you are calm inside, a simple thought can be absorbed by the subconscious mind and deeply integrated... can become a fundamental attitude, changing perception and experience, changing it to your advantage, because ear noises can become very, very quiet... and even disappear... So, you make yourself comfortable and, if you want, you can even wish to fall asleep... This way, you become even calmer, and everything disturbing falls asleep...

Now notice what you can feel or hear inside yourself... maybe the ear noises are not that loud now... or they are particularly clear because everything else is so quiet and harmonious... either you are connected to the noises or already behind them, because there it is quiet... You take a belief with you into your perception, a belief that you formulate... You say...

Behind all noises, it is quiet. I listen deeply within myself, deep into the silence and become free.

... [Read the affirmation slowly and a bit louder than the previous text to highlight it a bit. Then take a pause of about 30 seconds before continuing to read.] ...

And that is exactly what you do now... You listen deeply within yourself... sinking deeper and deeper into yourself... until you arrive behind the noises... maybe you are already behind the noises and have reached the silence... or your journey takes a little longer, and you are just moving through it and will arrive behind the noises in a few moments... But you will succeed... It really succeeds; you reach behind the ear noises, into the silence... either now or in a few moments, you are in the silence... This sentence, this helpful affirmation helps you... Affirmation means consolidation because this thought is supposed to and will consolidate...

This particular thought is your deep conviction... Conviction that you can use like a mantra and can think over and over again... or say it to further consolidate it... and let it become true again and again...

Behind all noises, it is quiet. I listen deeply within myself, deep into the silence and become free.

... Now take a breath... Let your breath flow, and deep inside, you will realize that you can really hear behind the noises... not just now in trance... You can do it whenever you want... You can do it in your waking everyday life... You can do it without thinking about it because it is a fundamental attitude, and you make sure that it remains your fundamental attitude... This is possible because that is exactly what affirmations are for... They are like little prayers or mantras... like a children's song that describes a truth... and ear noises become quieter and quieter, disappear...

So, let's go... It's time... You have already changed your own perspective deep inside... and you have changed your approach... can now deal with the ear noises completely differently... In trance, something like that is possible, and sometimes it's surprising how easy it then becomes... how easy it can be when you make an idea into a deep attitude in trance... and when this attitude suddenly becomes true... because you let a simple thought become true in you in a special way... it's a very simple thought, and you can tell yourself every day... you can repeat it to yourself three times a day because it is your thought, and your inner self is waiting for your daily affirmation... your thought is...

Behind all noises, it is quiet. I listen deeply within myself, deep into the silence and become free...

In a daily moment of reflection, you can close your eyes and repeat it... and if the ear noises consciously bother you, just close your eyes and repeat your belief... over and over again... and soon, annoying noises will disappear completely... You hear far behind them and thereby leave these noises behind you...

Hypnosis 5

You have made a decision... You want to end the disturbing ear noises... and there are two conceivable ways... They could disappear, or they could be transformed... Today, we are taking the path of transformation... because it is much easier to turn disturbing noises into pleasant ones... and then later, let them go entirely when it is so pleasant that you no longer need any other pleasant noises... Today, everything is supposed to be different... Today, all disturbing noises should become helpful noises... and that is indeed possible... maybe you wonder how quickly it can happen or how exactly it works... or maybe you already know deep inside...

We usually focus on the disturbing things and think about how to get rid of them... But there is another way, there is the possibility of dealing with the disturbing things differently... if it is possible to change something disturbing or to recognize something new in it, then it no longer disturbs... Imagine you could find something good in the ear noises... Imagine it wasn't a disturbance, and maybe it isn't really one... if the noises in the ear were like the sound of ocean waves on the shore, it would be different... The waves crashing on the shore might make a similar noise but calm you and are pleasant... The sound of waves brings you peace... that's easy... When you lie by the sea and close your eyes and hear the waves, it becomes quiet inside you... then you can even easily fall asleep because the sound of the waves calms you so much that you relax... that you really relax to this sound...

Now listen to yourself and hear the noise in your ear... hear the sound of the waves that calm you... Let yourself be calmed by the sound of the waves in your ear... which are getting quieter and quieter... Imagine being there... by the sea... and with your eyes closed, you lie there in the sand... The more you succeed in having this image of lying there in the sand and hearing the waves, the sooner it becomes quieter inside you... quieter inside you... so that all noises gradually become gentle waves... All noises become the sound of gentle waves, slowly and softly rolling out... and making you tired and calm... The noises become more and more background noise... further and further away from you... into the background, and you hear them quieter and quieter... very quiet and far away... very quiet and far away... Noises are just quiet waves on the shore... Noises are just quiet waves on the shore... This way, the noises in the ear become a pleasant sound of nature that is gently heard in the background and calms you... reminds you of the waves of the sea...

Imagine how it was when the ear noises bothered you... maybe a specific situation comes to mind or a typical situation... and imagine that in this situation, you only heard the gentle sound of waves that would have calmed you... that would have calmed you, just like today... The situation that was so annoying before becomes much more pleasant with the gentle sound of waves... What used to be a burden becomes more pleasant now... Imagine once again that you were there... back then, it was annoying ear noises, today, it's beautiful waves on the shore... that is much more pleasant... that is much more comfortable... The sound of waves is pleasant... The sound of waves is even beautiful because it brings you peace... lets you relax... Feel the relaxation now and stay in the image of the beach by the sea... Continue to imagine that you are there and hear the waves with your eyes closed, calming you and making you tired... very tired and quiet... Now it works... at least as an image, as a fantasy, because you can imagine that it is so or at least can be so... and what is possible in your imagination can also happen in your waking everyday life, maybe a little later or a little slower... but everything you can think of can also become reality... just as peace is possible now, peace is always possible in your waking state... just as noises now become beautiful noises, it is also possible in waking everyday life... today or tomorrow... or every day of your life for another moment...

But you can do much more than just having this important fantasy today... You can transform the previously disturbing noises into helpful sounds every day... Whenever the ear noises start to bother you, you can awaken the image of the waves on the shore within you... And thus, the noises help you relax and only hear them in the background... and better yet, your subconscious mind does most of this for you... and as soon as there could be disturbing noises, your subconscious mind, your deep inner self, sends you an image of the helpful waves on the shore... an image of your peace and relaxation by the shore... and a part of you remains active and awake... but at the same time, a part of you inside goes to this place of beautiful waves on the shore... and this part of you enjoys the far-away sound of gentle waves... waves that are pleasant...

Now feel the peace and nothing but the peace within you... Allow yourself to do absolutely nothing and not worry anymore because when a big step is accomplished, you may rest... and you have accomplished a big step... a very big step... You have transformed the noises in your ear... made them into waves, far away... into pleasant noises... so you may now rest and enjoy the waves... just enjoy...

Hypnosis 6

Today is a special day because today is the day when you can overcome the disturbing ear noises... These noises were not only annoying and disturbing, but they also kept you from something... They kept you from dealing with important things within yourself... It wasn't your fault; it couldn't have been otherwise... because how could you listen to yourself and hear your inner voice when it was always buzzing or humming or ringing... But today, it is possible to hear behind these noises because behind disturbing noises, there is always something that wants to be seen... something that can help you truly overcome these noises... This is really possible once you can listen behind the noises, look behind the scenes... I will guide you on this path today...

Deep within yourself, there is a place of special encounter... It is a place of silence, behind all noises... This place of silence lies in your subconscious, and maybe you thought that the subconscious cannot be easily reached... but it is possible... it is possible in trance, and you are in trance right now... in this quiet state, you can also encounter the parts of yourself that you usually cannot perceive... the path there leads through feeling because the place of silence is in your feelings... behind all noises... Ear noises can be like a wall, but behind this wall is the place of silence... You can reach there today... you can go through the wall of noises... simply listen deeply within yourself... and look deeply into yourself...

Focus on the noises in the ear... Yes, focus on them, precisely because they are so disturbing... Trust that there is an inner voice behind these noises... because there really is... maybe as an auditory voice, as a sound... or as a feeling and thought... but there is the inner voice behind the ear noises... So now try to hear what is behind these noises... and then it's like you are suddenly far behind these noises... far behind, so that you only hear them quietly... because this wall is still there, but you are focusing your attention behind this wall... far behind, because there, deep inside, you can encounter your inner voice... a voice that speaks to you... You are now fully encountering the voice that speaks to you...

The voice that speaks to you is your own voice... the voice that speaks to you is the voice within you... the voice that speaks to you is the voice that can tell you something about yourself... the voice that speaks to you is the voice that can lead you to your feelings and needs... it leads you into your feelings... and deep in your feelings lie all the solutions... Once you have truly encountered your deepest feelings, disturbing noises can also really go away... The voice greets you... It is glad that you are here... it is glad that you are listening behind the noises, that you have broken through this wall and are listening deeper... and going deeper... understanding deeper and being able to change everything deep inside... The voice wants to help you... it can only do that behind the noise... and now, at this moment, you have left the ear noises behind to listen and look deeper inside yourself... to be with your inner, helpful voice that speaks to you... The voice tells you about the burden of the ear noises, and you know this burden, you have experienced it yourself... The voice also tells you that these noises have helped you... They have burdened you, and maybe there is a physiological reason why they came, but they can also get quieter and slowly fade away... Your helpful voice explains that despite the suffering, you also had an advantage from the noises because you couldn't hear the inner voice that is now speaking to you... That was important, too, because it would have been too much to pay attention to the inner voice as well... You had a lot of stress and worries, had so many tasks to complete, that sometimes it would have been too much to deal with the inner voice as well... but today, it's possible... and here inside, something is waiting for you... something that wants to be heard... Maybe you already know what the inner voice wants to tell you... You now listen deeply within yourself because your inner voice wants to tell you something, and whatever it is that you can hear or think, just let it be until you hear my voice again... [Now please remain silent for about 30 seconds and then continue reading]...

... whatever the voice tells you, just let it be... because it is very important... whatever thought comes to you, it is a hint from your inner voice... You don't have to analyze or understand it, that's not the point... it only matters that you are there and listen to the voice, then the ear noises can get quieter and fade away... even if you couldn't hear anything or aren't sure what the voice wants to tell you, it will soon reach you... So the voice takes the ear noise with it, and you only take what the voice has told you, that's all you need... The noises go deep inside and fade there, so you no longer hear them... You only take with you what the inner voice has told you, and that leads to silence and peace...

Now you can come back, be present in the outside again... A new connection has been made... a connection from you to your inner voice, and this new connection can't be interrupted by any wall... because it is a deep connection from you to yourself... behind every noise...

Hypnosis 7

You are here today because you want to let go of your disturbing ear noises... you want to turn them off... to end this tinnitus... once and for all... and that is possible... because your body fundamentally follows your thoughts and feelings... and you can help your body to take a different direction... to make tinnitus noises quieter or to ignore them... especially when they are physiological and cannot be eliminated... You know this from everyday life... When you focus on something and are fully absorbed, you no longer hear other noises... When a thought fascinates you and you are engrossed in something, you might not even hear someone calling your name... Surely, you have experienced this before... So, you know that it really is true that attention and focus lead you to perceive certain noises, others less... or not hear them at all... You also don't always hear the ear noises at the same volume... sometimes, when you are very focused or with great joy engaged in something else, you don't pay attention to the tinnitus at all, don't hear it at all... You can actively control and influence something like that...

It's really possible... It's quite amazing, but it really is possible...

You can focus completely on my voice... You try it out and focus entirely on my voice... In doing so, you can make other noises quieter... The music in the background slowly fades... It's as if you're turning it down... My voice becomes clearer... You hear every word... You hear every sound very clearly... Everything else becomes unimportant and quiet... Isn't it amazing how you can direct your attention... and how quiet many noises become in the process... You can do even more... Now you focus on the music in the background... You direct your hearing toward the music... You try to hear it clearly... My voice becomes quieter and fades into the background... My voice slowly fades... step by step... The more you focus on the music, the quieter my voice becomes... It fades more and more and becomes unimportant... Only the music is important now... It's as if you are turning it up with your thoughts... You tune out all other noises... Isn't it amazing how you can direct your attention... and how quiet many noises become in the process... You can direct your attention and change the volume of the noises in your ear... Disturbing noises become quieter... They fade into the background... You direct your attention to the really important things... to my voice... to the music... because both are important now... You can hear both simultaneously and equally clearly... my voice and the music... All other noises become quieter... They fade into the background... Isn't it amazing how you can direct your attention... and how quiet many noises become in the process... You shift your attention outward... You direct your attention to the noises coming from outside... So now you perceive all the noises from the outside clearly... my voice and the music and maybe you find other sounds outside your body... There are more noises in this room... Isn't it amazing how you can direct your attention... and how quiet many noises become in the process... Shift your perception to the room we are in... Focus on all the noises here in the room and try to perceive other sounds besides my voice and the music... Focus your hearing and you will perceive more noises... All other noises inside you become quieter... You tune out all disturbing noises... Isn't it amazing how you can direct your attention... and how quiet many noises become in the process... Now shift your perception even further outside... Try to perceive noises outside the room... Go around the house in your mind and find sounds outside that you can hear... You focus entirely on hearing sounds outside the house... You can recognize some sounds... You let them become intense... As if you are standing in front of the house now and hearing everything outside... All the noises in the room become quieter and fade into the background... Even my voice becomes very quiet... Isn't it amazing how you can direct your attention... and how quiet many noises become in the process... Now let your hearing wander further and return entirely to yourself... You listen to yourself and feel that it has become quiet... much quieter than before... When your attention goes outward, it becomes quiet within you... The silence spreads within you when you return and listen to yourself... Isn't it amazing how you can direct your attention... and how quiet many noises become in the process...

Now you can let go of all thoughts because your body has long understood how it works... your body knows how to direct your attention so that you hear all the noises outside, but inside the ear, there are no more noises... Only the noises from outside reach you, only they can be heard clearly... Ear noises don't matter anymore... they only stay in the background... and move further and further into the background every day... so that you can no longer really perceive them... so that you don't notice the ear noises anymore... so that it becomes quiet in the ear... quiet and calm in your ear...

Hypnosis 8

Analytical Reframing Ideomotorics

Ideomotorics refers to the phenomenon that our body follows our feelings and thoughts with movements. In everyday life, this following is expressed as body posture, muscle tension, and movement patterns of a person, which naturally change with the mood and thoughts. In trance, ideomotor signals can be used to obtain information that the client cannot actively communicate. The subconscious can answer questions with an agreed-upon finger signal, for example. Of course, ideomotor responses can also be used suggestively, such as in arm levitations and catalepsies. An ideomotor approach strengthens trust in hypnosis and one's ability to change, thereby promoting therapy.

You want to make the ear noises disappear... at least they should become quieter today and then gradually fade away completely... That is possible because a special part of you can accomplish that... a part or aspect of you that you cannot consciously control in a waking state... but it is possible in trance because in trance, you are one with yourself, you can also reach and use the unconscious areas within you... Maybe you know that what burdens us is often a signal from this unconscious area within us... a signal that we are not feeling well inside and that we need to take care of ourselves... it's the same with ear noises that are disturbing and don't go away easily... but they can go away once you manage to connect with exactly these unconscious areas because then you are taking care of yourself... differently than before... Your subconscious cares about you connecting with it because then disturbing ear noises can be ended... This special part of you, the unconscious or subconscious, no longer needs a signal... no more ear noises... for this, I need to speak directly with your subconscious... Dream in beautiful images, imagine a beautiful landscape, as vividly as possible... and stay in the beautiful images of this landscape... so beautiful that you would love to be there... You can hear every word and feel everything, but just stay in your beautiful images and imagine that all thoughts and ideas, all beautiful images you think of, move to the left... to the left side of the body... and you, subconscious of... [client's first name]... come to the right and control the right hand... and give me a signal with a finger of the right hand once you have succeeded in taking control of the hand... While the waking consciousness dreams on the left side in beautiful images, you subconscious of... [client's first name]... come to the right and move a finger of the right hand...

... [Be patient and stick with it. Don't worry – finger signals (almost) always succeed! Repeat the request a few times kindly and with a bit of emphasis and exude confidence. If you are sure that a finger signal will come, it happens faster than if you doubt.] ...

... There is the signal, excellent... Thank you very much... Now, subconscious of... [client's first name]... make sure that the waking consciousness dreams deeply on the left side, so we can work well together... The welcoming finger should be the yes finger... for each confirmation, you can move it... for rejection, you can move another finger... but now we want to do what your goal is... understand and then end the ear noises... Now it begins...

Subconscious of... [client's first name]... we want to try to understand the ear noises better so that you can end them... because I know that you can and will do that if we carefully address them... For this, I will ask you some questions that you can answer with your fingers... for a yes, please use the yes finger and for a no, choose another finger... and for undecided, move the yes finger and another one at the same time...

... Do the ear noises still have a helpful function for you today?

... if yes... Then let this function now flow as an image into the waking consciousness

... if no... good, then it is even easier to end them...

... Did the ear noises have a meaning when they started?

... if yes... That time is over, today you can proceed differently and end them...

... if no... Then the noises belong to something completely different and are no longer appropriate...

... Is there a connection to childhood and events back then?

... if yes... That was long ago, so let's look at childhood and understand it, today you are an adult and no longer need ear noises from childhood...

... if no... That's good, because then the problem hasn't been around for too long, and we can solve it faster...

... Is there something about the ear noises that we haven't recognized yet?

... if yes... We need another way to see it, a pleasant one, so we can truly understand it together...

... if no... Then we have already talked about what is important to you... Let's keep looking at and addressing it without ear noises, they are no longer necessary now...

... Subconscious of... [client's name]... You recognize that we are making an effort together to recognize and understand you and help you... The waking consciousness and I... And we will continue to do so, and I promise you that the waking consciousness will continue to make an effort to understand your hints and messages... That is what the waking consciousness does for you... what you have to do is reduce the noises as much as possible, if possible also turn them off... Only if it cannot be otherwise or if the waking consciousness breaks its word, could you turn the ear noises back on... Agreed?

... ... [A no doesn't come here anymore]... Good, then now reduce the ear noises, arrange everything so that they become as quiet as possible or disappear in the next 24 hours, and show me with the yes finger when you are done... [wait for the yes finger]...

Good, it has succeeded... Now the ear noises can fade away... Maybe you already notice it, and it is already happening, or you will be happy in the next 24 hours that they are getting quieter and quieter... fading more and more into the background...

Hypnosis 9

Today you are learning a special kind of hypnosis... hypnosis that works very simply and is very effective when a few simple conditions are met... Maybe you are already wondering how it will be, are excited about it... or you are already looking forward to experiencing how quickly your ear noises can fade away because you previously thought they wouldn't be so easy to alleviate... So, you are preparing yourself to actually get rid of the ear noises very quickly, faster than you thought... Now it's all about it... You want it... You want to get rid of the ear noises, have been waiting a long time for them to stop... so now is the right time for it... Surely you expected that it could eventually succeed because that's why you're here, to do something to get rid of the noises... but it happens faster than you thought... much faster...

Today you don't have to do anything... and doing nothing means that you only follow a very simple, visual imagination... that you imagine a very simple picture that I will introduce to you in a few moments... Then you don't have to do anything else, you simply imagine the picture, and it happens automatically when I speak of it... It can't be otherwise; it can only happen and succeed because when I mention a picture, you automatically imagine it... at least for an important moment, which can be very short... It only matters to focus on your goal and then visualize the picture once... imagine it... as well as you can... The better you succeed in just looking at this picture, the faster you reach your goal... or more precisely: The goal reaches you... becomes true on its own... That simple? Yes... that simple...

Now focus on your goal just once... and then let go of every thought and focus only on a picture that I suggest to you... We will go through these two steps together... Ear noises belong to the past... only to the past... and so it shall be now and remain...

Fading out of ear noises, and freedom and silence within.

... [When pronouncing the goal formulation, feel free to place your palm on the client's solar plexus and then pull it away again. It is not necessary but helps a lot because the goal formulation is thereby "anchored." Of course, you can also incorporate energetic techniques into the hypnosis. Make sure not to repeat the goal.]...

Now imagine, with your eyes closed, that you are looking at a candle... Imagine the small, yellow flame... and imagine a direct connection from you to the candle... through your eyes... then suddenly it's as if you could hypnotize the candle... it only succeeds by looking directly into the flame and always keeping your gaze on it... until I tell you that you can let go of the picture again... Look into the flame and connect with the light... and imagine that you can control the flame with your thoughts... if you think to the left, the flame tilts to the left... continues to burn calmly, but tilted to the left... and if you think that it should burn straight again, the flame straightens up again... and now to the other side... Imagine tilting the flame to the right... it tilts to the right, continues to burn calmly and stably... tilted to the right... and again, you release the flame, and it straightens up... burns stably and straight... good... The connection is established, exists in your imagination, and thus in your subconscious... so you can tilt the burning flame to the left again... [wait about ten seconds]... and let it straighten up again... [wait about ten seconds]... and now to the right...

[wait about ten seconds]... and straighten up again... [wait about ten seconds]... and again and again, natural order is created when you let go in your mind... natural and calm order is always created... That's how it should be... a simple thought... a very simple image in you that brings your inner self into order... that ensures balance and harmony... That simple? Yes... that simple... and now feel the peace within you... and trust that with the inner order in your imagination, inner order in feeling and energy has also become possible... has actually already arisen and is unfolding... a beautiful, inner harmony... a very beautiful inner harmony...

So, the most important thing is done... because it doesn't take more than a goal and then freedom within yourself... freedom of your subconscious to get everything right... and exactly this freedom your subconscious has now had... in the short time of the image you have created... because whenever you focus entirely on a simple image, there are no disturbing thoughts... and your deep inner self, your subconscious, can freely put everything in order... also, and especially ensure that your ear noises can disappear because inner order and disturbing ear noises are not compatible...

So trust that the inner order continues, and as soon as it is sufficiently established, the ear noises fade away... very soon... Maybe even now or in a few moments... or you will be happy tomorrow that the ear noises have disappeared... because it will happen...

Hypnosis 10

In our imagination, we sometimes dream ourselves to the strangest places... Places that can't exist in the waking everyday life because space and time do not exist in imagination... we simply travel to the world of our imagination... a world where we can do everything and achieve everything we strive for... and then suddenly we realize that there are similarities between imagination and everyday life... because all ideas and wishes are formed by the truth within ourselves... by the truth of our feelings because only they are the source of our fantasies... what becomes true in the inner world, through a simple thought, a simple imagination... that can also become true in waking everyday life... a little different and a little slower, but the same truth... So now you go into this world of imagination within you... You go into the land of your dreams... and today you find a truth that begins anew...

You arrive in the land of dreams and look around... It is an autumn day, windy and cool... You are standing in a hilly landscape and can hear the wind blowing over the hills...

You look up, and the sky is gray... a gray autumn sky with many clouds... it looks like a storm is brewing because it is getting louder... the wind is blowing harder and whips up the leaves... whistles through the bare branches of the trees... Then you see a storm front coming toward you... like a wall slowly advancing, moving toward you... and you start walking... You walk toward the storm because in the land of dreams, you have the power... You can change everything and shape everything the way you want it here... Imagination changes everything here... and your imagination can end any rough storm... can make the rushing, lashing wind quiet... but you walk toward the storm because you want to see and experience it... because a voice tells you that you should go behind the storm... to where everything is calm... because behind the storm, there are no rough winds... no rushing and no stormy humming... Behind the storm, everything is quiet, but there is also more... You think about the ear noises and how they might have started... maybe you also know how they came, have an idea about it or a notion... or someone has explained to you why they are there... and yet you have the question of why they have not gone away... why your body hasn't been able to end this humming, rough wind in your ear yet... Behind the storm, you will find a new answer... So you walk directly toward the storm front...

It is like a gray wall coming toward you, and you walk toward it... a wall in the land of dreams... a wall of wind and storm noises... the same noises that are in your ear that you have known and carried with you for so long... You arrive at the storm wall that stops... and you probably hear the noises in your ear very clearly now... or they are entirely in the land of dreams and only there, at the storm wall, in front of which you stand... and because nothing can happen to you here, you walk into the storm... The wind pulls and tugs at you and tries to tear you away, but nothing can happen to you in the land of dreams... You keep walking and remember the storms of your life... Often, it was as if you fought in the storm and something or someone pulled at you from all sides... the events of life's storms threw you off balance, maybe even off course at times... but somehow you kept going, kept fighting... kept getting up again... even if you had fallen so painfully... and then it was as if an echo of life's storms remained in your ears... like a sound recording... a memory that kept playing, maybe because you couldn't imagine that the storms would end... But suddenly, in the land of dreams, it becomes quiet and calm... the wind fades away... You have walked through the storm wall... it's as if you have passed through a gate and arrived in a peaceful world... The sun is shining... you look up, the sky is blue, and there are no clouds... You are in a beautiful natural landscape, and it is a quiet, warm summer day... wonderful, so beautiful it is behind the storm wall... so calm it is behind every storm... You find a beautiful place to rest from the hardships of the past... maybe in the shade of a tree or simply in the sunshine... You set up a beautiful place of peace and find everything you need for it... maybe a hammock or a mattress... a soft blanket or thick pillows... a bench to sit on and enjoy the view once you've rested enough... to quietly look into the distance... to calmly overlook the dreamland and enjoy it... to quietly observe your thoughts and feelings and let them be there... because in the land of dreams, every thought and every feeling becomes images of nature... and no feeling can be bad or wrong... feelings are just there, and we can only accept them... fighting against them is like staying stuck in the storm and its stormy noises... Accepting feelings and turning them into images leads us back behind the storm front... to where there is simply peace...

You think about the land of dreams... consider what it might mean if you change something here, in the world of your own imagination... how it can help you get rid of your ear noises... or no longer be bothered by them... The land of dreams tells you that it's about feeling your own emotions... especially those that lie behind the anger and suffering, the feelings deep inside that want to be seen by you... and the land of dreams tells you that feelings can never be bad or wrong... actions can be wrong, but not feelings, because you can't control them... Accepting our own feelings is the key to ourselves... to peace after the storm... The land of dreams lies deep within you and has always been there... I'm just telling you about it...

Distribution, publication, and copying in any form are prohibited and subject to damages.

All Titles in the Series

Volume 1: Smoking Cessation
Volume 2: Anxiety and Restlessness
Volume 3: Burnout
Volume 4: Reducing Overweight
Volume 5: Coping with the Past
Volume 6: Suicidal Thoughts and Attempts
Volume 7: Psycho-Oncology
Volume 8: Obsessions and Tics
Volume 9: Self-Confidence and Decision-Making
Volume 10: Grief Work
Volume 11: Psychosomatics
Volume 12: Chronic Pain
Volume 13: Depressive Thoughts
Volume 14: Panic Attacks
Volume 15: Domestic Violence, Victim Support
Volume 16: Post-Traumatic Stress
Volume 17: Exam Anxiety and Stage Fright
Volume 18: Anti-Violence Training, Offender Support
Volume 19: Addiction Tendencies
Volume 20: Social Phobia and Fear of Contact
Volume 21: Nail Biting
Volume 22: Self-Awareness and Self-Love
Volume 23: Teeth Grinding and Night Clenching
Volume 24: Feelings of Guilt
Volume 25: Fear in Crowds
Volume 26: Fear of Flying, Aviophobia
Volume 27: Fear in Enclosed Spaces, Claustrophobia
Volume 28: Tinnitus, Ear Noises
Volume 29: Fear of Heights
Volume 30: Neurodermatitis

Copying, publishing, and sharing with third parties are only permitted with the written consent of the author. Please observe the notes on copyright and usage.

Volume 31: Finding Inner Balance
Volume 32: Overcoming Loneliness
Volume 33: Fear of Illness, Hypochondria
Volume 34: Anticipatory Anxiety, Fear of Fear
Volume 35: Jealousy in Relationships
Volume 36: Driving Anxiety
Volume 37: New Start after Separation
Volume 38: Fear of Injections
Volume 39: Heart Anxiety Neurosis
Volume 40: Overcoming Resentment and Anger
Volume 41: Resolving Blockages and Positive Thinking
Volume 42: Stress Reduction, Stress Management
Volume 43: Body Relaxation
Volume 44: Deep Relaxation
Volume 45: Fear of the Dark
Volume 46: Falling Asleep and Staying Asleep
Volume 47: Compulsive Buying
Volume 48: Restless Legs Syndrome
Volume 49: Bulimia
Volume 50: Anorexia
Volume 51: Overcoming Nightmares
Volume 52: Imagined Deformity
Volume 53: Overcoming Distrust, Finding Trust
Volume 54: Processing Failures
Volume 55: Humiliation, Emotional Hurt
Volume 56: Distressing Compassion, Vicarious Suffering
Volume 57: Self-Forgiveness
Volume 58: Self-Awareness, Self-Confidence
Volume 59: Saying No
Volume 60: Assertiveness
Volume 61: Setting Boundaries and Self-Assertion
Volume 62: Decision-Making Ability

Volume 63: Success Orientation
Volume 64: Ruminating, Circular Thinking
Volume 65: Accepting Pregnancy
Volume 66: Birth Preparation
Volume 67: Spiritual Opening
Volume 68: Joy of Life and Inner Lightness
Volume 69: Patience and Inner Peace
Volume 70: Fibromyalgia and Rheumatism
Volume 71: Irritable Bowel Syndrome, Crohn's Disease
Volume 72: Fear of Nausea, Emetophobia
Volume 73: Stuttering and Cluttering, Speech Flow Disorders
Volume 74: Concentration and Knowledge Anchoring
Volume 75: Vitality and Spontaneity
Volume 76: Searching for Meaning and Finding Goals
Volume 77: Life Crises, Life Events
Volume 78: Workaholism, Goal Obsession
Volume 79: Helper Syndrome, Helpless Helpers
Volume 80: Medication Abuse
Volume 81: Gambling Addiction
Volume 82: Internet Addiction, Smartphone Addiction
Volume 83: Hoarding Disorder, Compulsive Collecting
Volume 84: Conspiracy Thoughts, Overvalued Ideas
Volume 85: Fear of Operations and Treatments
Volume 86: Fear of Aging
Volume 87: Travel Anxiety
Volume 88: Anxiety When Urinating, Paruresis
Volume 89: Fear of Intimacy and Togetherness
Volume 90: Fear of Blushing
Volume 91: Coming Out in Homosexuality
Volume 92: Charisma Training
Volume 93: Migraines and Chronic Headaches
Volume 94: Overcoming Allergies, Bronchial Asthma

Volume 95: Normalizing Blood Pressure
Volume 96: Compulsive Perfectionism
Volume 97: Sports Hypnosis, Motivation
Volume 98: Sports Hypnosis, Performance Enhancement
Volume 99: Determination and Focus
Volume 100: Encountering the Inner Child
Volume 101: Cravings, Binge Eating
Volume 102: Stimulating Metabolism
Volume 103: Bipolar Mood Swings
Volume 104: Borderline, Identity Crises
Volume 105: Hypomania, Euphoria, Mania
Volume 106: Restlessness, Agitation
Volume 107: Nervous Breakdown
Volume 108: Adjustment Disorders
Volume 109: Self-Alienation, Depersonalization
Volume 110: Ending Self-Pity
Volume 111: Primary Gain of Illness
Volume 112: Secondary Gain of Illness
Volume 113: Bullying, Victim Support
Volume 114: Letting Go of Envy and Jealousy
Volume 115: Fear of Spiders, Arachnophobia
Volume 116: Fear of Dogs or Cats
Volume 117: Fear of Strangers, Xenophobia
Volume 118: Excessive Worries, Generalized Anxiety
Volume 119: Strengthening Sense of Responsibility
Volume 120: Unrequited Love, Heartache
Volume 121: Work-Life Balance
Volume 122: Letting Go of Unattainable Goals
Volume 123: Allowing and Accepting Help
Volume 124: Letting Go of Adult Children
Volume 125: Tourette Syndrome
Volume 126: Life Changes and New Starts

Volume 127: Accepting Life in a Wheelchair
Volume 128: Understanding and Overcoming Homesickness
Volume 129: Understanding and Overcoming Wanderlust
Volume 130: Dizziness, Meniere's Disease
Volume 131: Overcoming Aggression
Volume 132: Cutting and Self-Harm
Volume 133: Hair Pulling, Trichotillomania
Volume 134: Postpartum Depression
Volume 135: For Relatives of Dementia Patients
Volume 136: Self-Harm, Artificial Disorders
Volume 137: Activating Self-Healing Powers
Volume 138: Preventing Depression Relapse
Volume 139: Reactive Psychoses, Follow-Up
Volume 140: Obsessive Thoughts and Impulses
Volume 141: Compulsive Checking
Volume 142: Compulsive Counting, Symmetry Obsession
Volume 143: Compulsive Washing, Cleanliness Obsession
Volume 144: Compulsive Questioning
Volume 145: Dissociative Paralysis
Volume 146: Phantom Pain
Volume 147: Overcoming Complaining
Volume 148: Hay Fever, Pollen Allergy
Volume 149: Sexual Abuse, Victim Support
Volume 150: Standing Strong Against Sexism, #metoo
Volume 151: Binge Eating
Volume 152: Overcoming Thoughts of Revenge
Volume 153: Detachment from the Aggressor, Stockholm Syndrome
Volume 154: Courage to Separate
Volume 155: Chronic Fatigue, Exhaustion
Volume 156: Fear of the Future, Existential Anxiety
Volume 157: Excessive Worry About Children
Volume 158: Fear of Failure

Volume 159: Ending Distrust and Control
Volume 160: Dejection, Dysphoria
Volume 161: Boreout, Chronic Boredom
Volume 162: Bipolar Disorders, Relapse Prevention
Volume 163: Mania, Relapse Prevention
Volume 164: Nihilism, Feelings of Worthlessness
Volume 165: Thumb Sucking
Volume 166: Being Brave
Volume 167: Being Proud
Volume 168: Overcoming Shyness
Volume 169: Being Able to Delegate Responsibility
Volume 170: Being Able to Show Emotions
Volume 171: Letting Go of Guilt, Victim Support
Volume 172: Processing Guilt, Offender Support
Volume 173: Mood Swings, Cyclothymia
Volume 174: Lack of Drive, Vital Sadness
Volume 175: Hearing Voices with Reality Reference
Volume 176: Confident Communication
Volume 177: Standing Up for Oneself
Volume 178: Taking New Paths
Volume 179: Confident Job Application
Volume 180: No Longer Being Taken Advantage Of
Volume 181: End of Submissiveness
Volume 182: Depressive Numbness
Volume 183: Mood Drops, Affective Incontinence
Volume 184: Mood Instability
Volume 185: Somatoform Disorders
Volume 186: Stomach Ulcer, Psychosomatic
Volume 187: Accepting Amputation
Volume 188: Overcoming and Letting Go of Hatred
Volume 189: Ending Accusations
Volume 190: Allowing Tears, Being Able to Cry

Volume 191: Finding and Sorting Repressed Feelings
Volume 192: Somatoform Pain
Volume 193: Living Autonomously
Volume 194: Anhedonia, Joylessness
Volume 195: Persistent Sadness
Volume 196: Obesity, Food Addiction
Volume 197: Parents of Abused Children
Volume 198: Letting Go and Letting Be
Volume 199: Childhood Sexual Abuse
Volume 200: Fear of Loss

www.ingramcontent.com/pod-product-compliance
Lightning Source LLC
Chambersburg PA
CBHW030503220526
45464CB00006B/2628